Veröffentlichungen aus der
Geomedizinischen Forschungsstelle
(Leiter: Professor Dr. Dr. h.c. mult. G. Schettler)
der Heidelberger Akademie der Wissenschaften

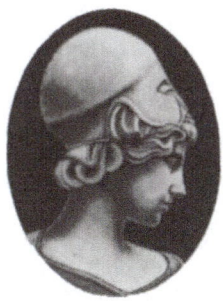

Supplement zu den Sitzungsberichten der
Mathematisch-naturwissenschaftlichen Klasse
Jahrgang 1988

G. Schettler (Ed.)

Recent Results of Research on Arteriosclerosis

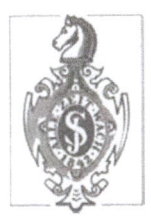

Springer-Verlag Berlin Heidelberg GmbH

Prof. Dr. Dr. h. c. mult. Gotthard Schettler
Präsident der Heidelberger Akademie der Wissenschaften
Karlstraße 4, D-6900 Heidelberg

ISBN 978-3-540-50288-3   ISBN 978-3-642-83605-3 (eBook)
DOI 10.1007/978-3-642-83605-3

Typesetting: K+V Fotosatz GmbH, Beerfelden
Printing and Binding: Druckhaus Beltz, Hemsbach/Bergstraße
2125/3140-543210 — Printed on acid-free paper

Contents

List of Contributors

Augustin, J., Prof. Dr.
Bereich Medizin, Merckle GmbH
Postfach 1780, 7900 Ulm-Donautal, FRG

Buchholz, L., Dr.
Abteilung Arbeitssicherheit,
Verwaltung des Klinikums der Universität Heidelberg
Voßstraße 1, 6900 Heidelberg, FRG

Goerig, M., Dr.
Abteilung Innere Medizin, Universität Heidelberg
Bergheimerstraße 58, 6900 Heidelberg, FRG

Grulich-Henn, J., Dr.
Max-Planck-Gesellschaft, Klinische Forschungsgruppe für
Blutgerinnung und Thrombose
Gaskystraße 11, 6300 Gießen, FRG

Habenicht, A., PD. Dr.
Abteilung Innere Medizin, Universität Heidelberg
Bergheimerstraße 58, 6900 Heidelberg, FRG

Haberbosch, W., Dr.
Abteilung Innere Medizin, Universität Heidelberg
Bergheimerstraße 58, 6900 Heidelberg, FRG

Morgenstern, W., Dipl.-Math.
Abteilung Klinische Sozialmedizin, Universität Heidelberg
Bergheimerstraße 58, 6900 Heidelberg, FRG

Nüssel, F.-E., Prof. Dr.
Abteilung Klinische Sozialmedizin, Universität Heidelberg
Bergheimerstraße 58, 6900 Heidelberg, FRG

Schettler, G., Prof. Dr. Dr. h. c. mult.
Geomedizinische Forschungsstelle, Heidelberger Akademie
der Wissenschaften
Karlstraße 4, 6900 Heidelberg, FRG

The Eberbach/Wiesloch Study: Influence of Cigarette Smoking on Lipoprotein Profiles

J. Augustin, J. Grulich-Henn, W. Haberbosch, L. Buchholz,
W. Morgenstern, F.-E. Nüssel, and G. Schettler

Summary

Plasma lipid and lipoprotein profiles, plasma cotinine levels, and smoking habits
of a randomly selected sample of middle-aged men and women in two representative towns of the Federal Republic of Germany were investigated. Mean plasma
cholesterol and triglyceride levels were significantly higher in smoking men and
women. Smoking women had significantly reduced high-density lipoprotein
(HDL) cholesterol levels. Smokers of both sexes had 16- to 20-fold higher plasma
cotinine levels than non- or ex-smokers. Plasma cotinine levels correlated
positively with very-low-density lipoprotein (VLDL) triglycerides, VLDL-
cholesterol, intermediate-density lipoprotein (IDL) triglycerides, low-density
lipoprotein (LDL) triglycerides, VLDL-apoprotein (Apo) CI, and HDL_3-Apo
CII in men and women. Positive correlations between plasma cotinine and Apo
CII, Apo $CIII_1$, and Apo $CIII_2$ of VLDL were only observed in women. On the
other hand, plasma cotinine correlated negatively with HDL_2 cholesterol, HDL_2
phospholipids, and HDL_2 Apo $CIII_1$ in both sexes. Futhermore, in women,
plasma cotinine correlated negatively with HDL_2 APO AI, HDL_2 APO AII,
HDL_2 Apo CI, HDL_2 Apo CII, and HDL_2 Apo $CIII_0$.

These results suggest that chronic cigarette smoking has profound effects on
plasma lipid and lipoprotein profiles, which become much more evident when
plasma cotinine levels are used as a quantitative parameter for cigarette consumption. Plasma cotinine seems a reliable and objective parameter to study the
influence of smoking habits. Finally, lipoprotein profiles of men and women are
affected differently.

Introduction

Smoking is one of the major risk factors for the development of atherosclerotic
cardiovascular disease [16, 17]. Numerous epidemiological studies have revealed
that mortality from ischemic heart attack is twice as high in smokers as in non-
smokers [3 – 7, 14, 18]. Despite the extensive data showing that smoking is a risk
factor, it is still unclear how smoking acts biologically to influence the development of atherosclerosis. Several studies have reported that smoking affects

plasma lipid and lipoprotein metabolism [9, 12, 13]. For example, heavy smokers had higher cholesterol and triglyceride levels, and smokers had significantly lower high-density lipoprotein (HDL) cholesterol levels than nonsmokers [2, 19]. However, plasma lipids and lipoproteins are also influenced by several other factors, e.g., sex, age, exercise, obesity, pill formulation, and alcohol intake. Cigarette smokers have been reported to be less obese, to exercise less, and to consume more alcohol [20]. Furthermore, the number of cigarettes smoked per day is not a very good quantitative measure of the consumption of tobacco ingredients. The number of cigarettes smoked per day may be over- or underestimated by the subjects investigated, the degree of inhalation may vary between individuals, and ingredients of cigarette smoke inhaled depend on the kind of tobacco and on filters that may be used.

In previous studies, we investigated the acute effects of cigarette smoking on lipoprotein metabolism [1]. We found an accelerated interconversion of triglyceride-rich very-low-density lipoproteins (VLDL) into low-density lipoproteins (LDL), a decrease in total HDL, and a relative increase in HDL_2 due to a decrease in HDL_3. Similar effects on lipoprotein metabolism were observed with nicotine-containing chewing gum, suggesting that the effects of smoking on plasma lipoproteins are mainly, if not completely, due to nicotine. These results were obtained under experimental conditions, and it is not known whether cigarette smokers have chronic alterations in lipoprotein metabolism which may have effects on the cardiovascular system. In the present study, we therefore investigated the lipid and lipoprotein profiles of smokers, nonsmokers, and exsmokers in a random sample of middle-aged men and women in two representative towns of the Federal Republic of Germany, and we compared lipid and lipoprotein levels with plasma cotinine, the main metabolite of nicotine.

Methods

Study Population. The study was conducted in connection with a Cardiovascular Comprehensive Community Control Programme (CCCCP) initiated by the World Health Organisation (WHO) [15]. In 1975, the WHO Collaborating Center in Heidelberg started a survey in Eberbach and Wiesloch, two towns near Heidelberg. The size of these towns and the age and sex distribution of the inhabitants are representative of about two-thirds of the population in the Federal Republic of Germany. In 1975, the population of 30- to 49-year-old men and women in Eberbach and Wiesloch consisted of 9908 people. In 1976/1977 a baseline screening was performed in which 98% of this sample were examined. A 10% random sample of those people aged 30 – 44 years in 1976/1977 was reexamined in 1981/1982. The present study was performed within that reexamination. The study group consisted of 237 men and 216 women aged 35 – 49 years. Of the men, 92 were smokers, 74 nonsmokers, and 71 exsmokers. Of the women, 56 were smokers, 136 nonsmokers, and 20 exsmokers.

Examination Procedures. The study involved two separate examinations of the participants. The first consisted of a home visit, where the blood samples were taken after a 12-h fasting period (usually in the morning). The blood withdrawal was done by trained personnel following a highly standardized procedure. The whole home visit usually took place within 10 minutes. A date for the second examination, at the practice of a local physician, was arranged. The second examination consisted of a standardized questionnaire and a physical examination, which included measurement of blood pressure, body height, and body weight.

Measurement of plasma lipids. Plasma cholesterol, triglycerides and phospholipids were measured using commercially available kits (Boehringer, Mannheim, FRG).

Lipoprotein Separation and Quantification. Lipoproteins were separated by preparative ultracentrifugation, as previously described [8]. EDTA blood was centrifuged for 30 min at 2500 rpm (4 °C) in a Beckman J6B centrifuge. Of the plasma obtained, 10 ml was filled into Beckman Quick Seal tubes (16 × 76 mm), overlaid with 0.9% NaCl, and centrifuged for 22 h at 50000 rpm (4 °C) in a Beckman L8-70 preparative ultracentrifuge, using a Beckman 70.1 Ti rotor. VLDL were obtained by slicing the tubes at 4 cm. The infranatant was adjusted to a density of 1.019 g/ml by addition of KBr and centrifuged for 22 h as described above to separate intermediate-density lipoproteins (IDL). LDL and HDL subfractions (HDL_2 and HDL_3) were obtained by additional ultracentrifugation steps at densities of 1.063 g/ml, 1.125 g/ml, and 1.210 g/ml, respectively. The densities were controlled by a Heraeus-Paar DMA 45 Densitometer. The height at which the tubes were sliced was obtained empirically by measuring the densities and performing lipid electrophoresis and zonal ultracentrifugation of the fractions.

VLDL, IDL, and LDL were perfectly separated from each other. There was a slight overlap between HDL_2 and HDL_3. The lipoproteins with a density of 1.063 g/ml contained about 2% albumin, while albumin represented 4% − 8% of the total protein bulk in HDL_2 and HDL_3. HDL were free of apoprotein (Apo) B. In the lipoprotein-free plasma (1.21 g/ml infranatant), 4% − 6% of total triglycerides, 3% − 4% of total cholesterol, and about 5% of the different apoproteins were found. An aliquot of each fraction was used to determine the lipid concentration, and the remaining fractions were dialyzed against distilled water (Visking Dialysis Tubing, type 8/32, Serva, Heidelberg, FRG) and lyophilized. The samples were then delipidated with 2 × 5 ml ethanol/ether (3 : 1, v/v) for 20 and 4 h, respectively, and finally with 5 ml ether for 1 h at − 18 °C.

Isoelectric focusing on ultrathin flat gels (0.3 mm) was used for separation and quantification of the apoproteins [8, 10]. The gels were prepared as follows: a 7% acrylamide solution with 2% ampholynes (pH 4 − 6 or 6 − 8, Serva, Heidelberg, FRG) was polymerized on plastic sheets. Anolyte and catholyte were 0.5 *M*

H_3PO_4 and 0.4 M NaOH, respectively. After a prerun for about 1 h to allow the formation of the pH gradient, 20 µl delipidated proteins dissolved in urea, Tris HCl pH 8.3 (7 mol/liter), was applied to the plate using rubber wells. Focusing time was 3 h at 1000 V, amperage free. Then the protein bands were fixed for 10 min with 10% trichloroacetic acid and 5 min with 7% acetic acid. The gels were stained for 15 min in 1% Light Green (Serva, Heidelberg, FRG) and then destained for 3×10 min with 7% acetic acid. The density of the stained bands was determined by an LKB 2202 Ultra Scan Laser Densitometer and compared with that of standards of known concentrations. Purified apoproteins, used as standards, were obtained from plasma of normal subjects for Apo AI and Apo AII, or hypertriglyceridemic subjects for C peptides, by gel filtration, affinity chromatography, and preparative isoelectric focusing. The purity of the apoproteins was controlled with excess amounts of proteins by SDS gel electrophoresis and isoelectric focusing. In addition, no cross-reactivity with antibodies against other apoproteins was observed. Standard curves were performed with every isolated apoprotein. When the concentration of the sample was not in the rectilinear part of the standard curve, it was diluted to achieve an appropriate concentration. The CIII isoforms showed identical chromogenicity, which was, however, different from Apo CI and Apo CII. The assay variations for Apo AI, AII, CI, CII, and CIII were 3.73%, 2.64%, 2.19%, 2.37%, and 1.44%, respectively. Apo B was determined by immunodiffusion on NOR partigen plates (Behringwerke AG, Marburg, FRG).

Measurement of Cotinine. Continine, a degradation product of nicotine, was measured by gas liquid chromatography, as previously described [11].

Quality Control. The study procedures were carried out according to the WHO guidelines. Established internal quality controlly procedures were used in the laboratory to ensure high levels of precision and accuracy for the lipid and lipoprotein determination. External quality controls were performed by the WHO Lipid Reference Laboratory, Europe (Dr. Grafnetter, Prague), and in cooperation with the reference laboratory of Boehringer Co., Mannheim.

Data Handling and Statistical Analysis. The data were recorded in a database system that has been developed by the Abteilung für Klinische Sozialmedizin at the University of Heidelberg. Before further analysis was performed, an error-screening program was used to find and eliminate incorrect data inputs. The statistical analysis was done using SAS (Statistical Analysis System, SAS Institute Inc., Cray, NC).

Results

Table 1 shows that smokers of both sexes had higher plasma cholesterol and triglyceride levels than non-smokers. Male ex-smokers also had significantly higher

Table 1. Plasma lipids and smoking habits

	Level (mg/dl)		
	Smokers	Non-smokers	Ex-smokers
Men			
Cholesterol	237.67[a]	225.28	237.86[a]
Triglycerides	268.40[a]	202.55	226.20
Phospholipids	292.33	297.96	308.71
HDL-cholesterol	51.86	53.22	54.56
Women			
Cholesterol	217.88[a]	207.86	199.60
Triglycerides	133.56[a]	104.09	107.50
Phospholipids	282.15	268.12	297.63
HDL-cholesterol	58.66[a]	64.46	68.90

[a] Significantly different from non-smokers ($P < 0.05$).

Table 2. Plasma cotinine and smoking habits

		Mean level (ng/ml)			
	n	Mean	25%	50%	75%
Men					
Smokers	89	150.2	50.0	122.0	176.5
Non-smokers	70	9.1	0.0	2.5	8.0
Ex-smokers	61	7.4	0.0	1.0	9.0
Women					
Smokers	53	89.4	24.5	74.0	147.0
Non-smokers	129	4.8	0.0	0.0	7.5
Ex-smokers	20	6.0	0.0	0.0	6.7

plasma cholesterol levels. Significantly lower HDL cholesterol levels were found in smoking women, but not in smoking men.

In order to investigate influences of smoking habits on lipoprotein profiles, we measured apolipoprotein and lipid levels in all lipoprotein classes and compared them with plasma cotinine levels. Table 2 shows that mean plasma cotinine levels in smokers were 16- to 20-fold higher than those in non- and ex-smokers. Mean and median cotinine levels in men were about 50% higher than those in women, suggesting that more men are heavy smokers than women (Table 2). We do not know whether the plasma cotinine levels between 6 and 9 ng/ml found in

Table 3. Correlation between plasma cotinine and lipoprotein fractions in men (Spearman correlation coefficients)

Apoprotein	VLDL	IDL	LDL	HDL$_2$	HDL$_3$
AI				NS	−0.14[a]
AII				NS	NS
B	NS	NS	NS		
CI	0.18[b]	NS	NS	NS	NS
CII	NS	NS	NS	NS	0.17[a]
CIII$_0$	NS	NS	NS	−0.13[a]	−0.13[a]
CIII$_1$	NS	NS	NS	NS	NS
CIII$_2$	NS	NS	NS	NS	NS
E	NS	NS	NS	NS	NS
Cholesterol	0.16[a]	NS	NS	−0.18[b]	−0.23[c]
Triglycerides	0.14[a]	0.15[a]	0.18[b]	NS	0.16[a]
Phospholipids	NS	NS	NS	−0.18[b]	NS

NS, no significant correlation.
[a] $P < 0.05$.
[b] $P < 0.01$.
[c] $P < 0.001$.

Table 4. Correlations between plasma cotinine and lipoprotein fractions in women (Spearman correlation coefficients)

Apoprotein	VLDL	IDL	LDL	HDL$_2$	HDL$_3$
AI				−0.22[b]	NS
AII				−0.15[a]	NS
B	NS	NS	NS		
CI	0.26[c]	NS	NS	−0.15[a]	0.20[b]
CII	0.23[b]	NS	NS	NS	0.20[b]
CIII$_0$	NS	NS	NS	−0.20[b]	NS
CIII$_1$	0.14[a]	NS	NS	−0.16[a]	NS
CIII$_2$	0.14[a]	NS	NS	NS	NS
E	NS	NS	NS	NS	NS
Cholesterol	0.18[b]	NS	NS	−0.22[b]	NS
Triglycerides	0.20[b]	0.16[a]	0.17[a]	NS	0.20[b]
Phospholipids	NS	0.19[b]	NS	−0.23[b]	NS

NS, no significant correlation.
[a] $P < 0.05$.
[b] $P < 0.01$.
[c] $P < 0.001$.

25% – 50% of non- and ex-smokers are due to passive smoking or represent occasional smokers who claimed to be non-smokers.

Positive correlations between plasma cotinine and VLDL Apo CI, VLDL cholesterol, and VLDL triglycerides were observed in both sexes. In women, there were also positive correlations between cotinine and VLDL Apo CII, VLDL Apo $CIII_1$, and VLDL Apo $CIII_2$. Positive correlations between cotinine levels on the one hand and IDL- and LDL triglycerides on the other hand were seen in men and women (Tables 3, 4). Negative correlations between cotinine and most of the HDL_2 fractions were observed in women. Interestingly, in HDL_2 profiles of men, only AP $CIII_0$, cholesterol, and phospholipids showed significant negative correlations with cotinine. Negative correlations between cotinine and HDL_3 Apo AI, HDL_3 Apo $CIII_0$, and HDL_3 cholesterol were only observed in men (Table 3).

It is well known that besides sex, age and obesity are independently related to plasma lipids and lipoproteins. Within the age group investigated, there were no age-specific differences in lipoprotein profiles, probably because the age intervals were not that big. In order to eliminate the influence of body mass on the correlations between plasma cotinine and lipoprotein profiles, partial correlation procedures matched on Broca index (body weight $\times 100$/body height $- 100$) were performed. Table 5 shows that in men several of the significant correlations observed with the Spearman procedure (Table 3) disappeared. However there was still a significant positive correlation between cotinine and LDL triglycerides, and a significant negative correlation between cotinine and HDL_3 cholesterol.

Table 5. Plasma cotinine and lipoproteins in men (partial correlation procedure matched on Broca index)

Apoprotein	VLDL	IDL	LDL	HDL_2	HDL_3
AI				NS	NS
AII				NS	NS
B	NS	NS	NS		
CI	NS	NS	NS	NS	NS
CII	NS	NS	NS	NS	NS
$CIII_0$	NS	NS	NS	NS	NS
$CIII_1$	NS	NS	NS	NS	NS
$CIII_2$	NS	NS	NS	NS	NS
E	NS	NS	NS	NS	NS
Cholesterol	NS	NS	NS	NS	-0.14[a]
Triglycerides	NS	NS	0.16[b]	NS	NS
Phospholipids	NS	NS	NS	NS	NS

NS, no significant correlation.

[a] $P < 0.05$.

[b] $P < 0.01$.

Table 6. Plasma cotinine and lipoproteins in women (partial correlation procedure matched on Broca index)

Apoprotein	VLDL	IDL	LDL	HDL$_2$	HDL$_3$
AI				−0.14[a]	NS
AI				−0.14[a]	NS
B	NS	NS	NS		
CI	0.24[c]	NS	NS	NS	0.13[a]
CII	0.26[c]	NS	NS	−0.15[a]	NS
CIII$_0$	0.13[a]	0.10[a]	NS	NS	NS
CIII$_1$	0.20[b]	NS	NS	−0.14[a]	NS
CIII$_2$	0.17[a]	NS	NS	−0.13[a]	NS
E	NS	NS	NS	NS	NS
Cholesterol	0.26[c]	0.16[b]	NS	−0.16[b]	NS
Triglycerides	0.26[c]	0.14[a]	0.14[a]	NS	0.15[a]
Phospholipids	NS	NS	NS	−0.15[a]	NS

NS, no significant correlation.
[a] $P < 0.05$.
[b] $P < 0.01$.
[c] $P < 0.001$.

In women only minor differences were seen between the partial correlation procedure matched on Broca index (Table 6) and the simple Spearman correlation procedure (Table 4). The correlation between cotinine and HDL$_2$ Apo CI, HDL$_2$ Apo CIII$_0$, and HDL$_3$ Apo CII disappeared. However, significant correlations between cotinine and IDL Apo CI, IDL Apo CIII0, IDL cholesterol, and HDL$_2$ Apo CIII$_2$, which had not been significant using the Sperman correlation procedure, became evident (Table 6). The correlation coefficient for VLDL cholesterol and VLDL triglycerides in women was higher when the partial correlation procedure was used (Tables 4, 6).

Discussion

Several studies have described associations between cigarette smoking and alterations in plasma lipid levels. Cigarette smoke contains a mixture of thousands of different compounds, and it is not known which components are responsible for the deleterious effects. In the present study, we investigated lipid and lipoprotein profiles in middle-aged smokers, non-smokers, and ex-smokers. The data presented here show the following distinct alterations in lipid and lipoprotein metabolism of smokers:

1. Smokers of both sexes had higher plasma cholesterol and triglyceride levels than non-smokers (Table 1). These data are consistent with previous studies which

reported higher cholesterol and triglyceride levels in heavy smokers [2, 9, 13, 19]. Several studies described an inverse relationship between cigarette smoking and HDL cholesterol levels. In the present study, HDL cholesterol was significantly decreased only in smoking women (Table 1).

2. Correlations of plasma cotinine levels and lipoprotein fractions displayed several significant links. Positive correlations were observed in VLDL, IDL, and LDL fractions (Tables 3, 4). Negative correlations were observed in HDL_2 fractions (Tables 3, 4). More significant correlations between cotinine and lipoprotein fractions were observed in women. In order to correct for the influence of body mass on lipoproteins, a partial correlation procedure matched on Broca index was performed. In men, most of the significant correlations shown in Table 3 disappeared when this procedure was used (Table 5). However, only minor changes were observed in women with this correlation procedure (Table 6). Thus, the correlations between cotinine and lipoprotein fractions in men were influenced by body mass. On the other hand, in women the correlations observed were scarcely influenced by body mass. Cotinine is the main metabolite of nicotine, and it can be detected in plasma even after weeks. It thus serves as an excellent marker for cigarette consumption.

In previous studies, we reported similar effects of cigarette smoking and nicotine-containing chewing gum on plasma lipoproteins, suggesting that the alterations in lipoprotein metabolism are mainly due to nicotine [1]. However, these studies investigated acute effects of cigarette smoking and nicotine-containing chewing gum on lipoproteins, and it was not known whether these observations are relevant for alterations in lipid and lipoprotein profiles in chronic smokers. The results presented here suggest that cigarette smoking has chronic effects on lipid and lipoprotein metabolism. Furthermore, the data suggest that the alterations are mainly, if not only, due to nicotine consumption. We do not know why lipoprotein profiles of women are more affected than those of men. Women have in general more favorable lipoprotein profiles than men; in smoking women, the profiles show a trend towards the profiles of men. One explanation could be that smoking affects some protective factors (e.g., hormone regulation) in women. Unfortunately, we have no data on the sex hormone status of the study population. Other factors like occupation, socioeconomic class, exercise, or alcohol consumption were not addressed in this study, although we are aware of their importance.

In summary, our data indicate that smoking has an important impact on lipoprotein profiles, which is most likely mediated by nicotine. Furthermore, plasma cotinine levels seem to be a reliable parameter for investigating smoking habits.

Acknowledgements. The excellent technical assistance of I. Geldmacher, E. Glatting, M. Miltner, and D. Schraube is gratefully acknowledged. We further wish to thank C. Borrmann for her assistance in preparing the manuscript.

References

1. Augustin J, Beedgen B, Spohr U, Winkel F (1982) The influence of smoking on the plasmalipoproteins. Inn Med 9:104–108
2. Carlson LA, Boettiger LE (1972) Ischaemic heart disease in relation to fasting values of plasma triglyceride and cholesterol. Lancet 1: 865–868
3. Department of Health and Human Services (1983) The health consequences of smoking: cardiovascular disease. A report of the surgeon general. Rockville, MD
4. Doll R, Peto R (1976) Mortality in relation to smoking: 20 years observations on male British doctors. Br Med J 2:1525–1536
5. Doyle JT, Dawber TR, Kannel WB, Heslin AS, Kahn HA (1962) Cigarette smoking and coronary heart disease. N Engl J Med 266:796
6. Doyle JT, Dawber TR, Kannel WB, Kinch SH, Kahn HA (1964) The relationship of cigarette smoking to coronary heart disease. JAMA 190:108
7. Fielding JE (1985) Smoking: Health Effects on Control. N Engl J Med 313:491–498
8. Gnasso A, Lehner B, Haberbosch W, Leiss O, von Bergmann L, Augustin J (1986) Effects of Gemofibrozil on lipids, apoproteins, and postheparin lipolytic activities in normolipidemic subjects. Metabolism 35:387–393
9. Gofman JW, Lindgren FT, Strisower B, de Lalla O, Glazier F, Tamplin A (1955) Cigarette smoking, serum lipoproteins and coronary heart disease. Geriatrics 10:349
10. Haberbosch W, Poli A, Marx A, Augustin J (1982) Quantification of Apoproteins – Clinical Significance. Inn Med 9:99–103
11. Hengen N, Hengen M (1978) Gas liquid chromatographic determination of nicotine and cotinine in plasma. Clin. Chem. 24:50–55
12. Kershbaum A, Bellet S, Khorsandian R (1965) Elevation of serum cholesterol after administration of nicotine. Am Heart J 69:206–210
13. Kershbaum A, Bellet S (1968) Cigarette, cigar and pipe smoking. Geriatrics 23:126
14. Paul O, Lepper MH, Phelan WH, Dupertuis GW, Macmillan A, McKean H, Park H (1963) Coronary heart disease in industrial population: prospective Study. Circulation 28:20–31
15. Pisa Z, Strasser T (1981) Comprehensive cardiovascular control programme in the Community. WHO Europe, Copenhagen. Public Health Eur 5:101–114
16. Schettler G (1978) Die Ätiologie der Arteriosklerose. Der Internist 19:611–620
17. Schettler G, Gotto AM, Middelhoff G, Habenicht AJR, Jurutka KR (eds) Atherosclerosis VI. Springer, Berlin Heidelberg New York, pp 873–910 ("Smoking and atherosclerosis")
18. Spain DM, Nathan DJ (1961) Smoking habits and coronary artherosclerotic heart disease. JAMA 177:683–688
19. Wirth A (1982) Beeinflussung koronarer Risikofaktoren durch körperliches Training. Inn Med 9:130–133
20. Wynder EL, Hoffmann D, Gori GB (1975) Smoking and health. Proceedings of the 3rd World Conference. Modifying the Risk for the Smoker. DHEW Publ No (NIH) 76-1221

Fish Oil and Occlusive Vascular Disease*

M. Goerig, A. Habenicht, and G. Schettler

Summary

Fish oils and ω-3 polyunsaturated fatty acids exhibit hypolipidemic effects and both antiaggregatory and antiinflammatory properties (Table 1), they may lead to complex and only partially understood alterations of cellular interactions. The available data raise the question of the potential therapeutic and preventive value of dietary supplementation with ω-3 polyunsaturated fatty acids in occlusive vascular diseases.

Table 1. Properties of diets enriched with fish-oil-derived fatty acids

Hypolipidemic effects
Antiaggregatory effects
Antiinflammatory effects

Atherogenesis

The pathophysiology of atherosclerosis is a complex biological process that involves severe perturbations in cellular interactions and both lipoprotein and arachidonic acid metabolism. A wide variety of cell types produce distinct hormonal and humoral factors which serve as endogenous signals and regulate proliferation and differentiation of target cells, as well as immunological and inflammatory responses. Monocytes, platelets, endothelial cells, and smooth muscle cells exhibit critical interactions which have been suggested to be a prerequisite for the development of arteriosclerotic lesions [43, 96]. Deposition of clusters of monocytes on the arterial endothelium, migration of monocytes into the subendothelium, and subsequent transformation into foam cells appear to be the initial steps in atherogenesis. Retraction of the overlying endothelium, i.e.,

* This work was supported by the Forschungsrat Rauchen und Gesundheit, Hamburg, and the Deutsche Forschungsgemeinschaft (grants Ha 1083/3 – 1 and Ha 1083/2 – 3).

loss of endothelial continuity, permits platelet adherence and activation and may lead consecutively to mural and intramural thrombosis. Secretion of the potent mitogenic and chemotactic platelet-derived growth factor (PDGF), platelet factor 4, β-thrombomodulin, and products of the PGH synthase (cyclo-oxygenase) and 5-lipoxygenase pathways may contribute to the thrombotic process [86]. Proliferation of smooth muscle cells, their migration into the intima, and intracellular accumulation of lipids characterize fibrous plaque formation [96].

PDGF is synthesized and released not only by activated platelets but also by monocytes, endothelial cells, or (embryonal) smooth muscle cells, and it binds to specific receptors of target cells such as monocytes, polymorphonuclear leuko-cytes (PMN), smooth muscle cells, and fibroblasts. It is important to consider that PDGF is able both to provoke full expression of the entire PMN activation response and to promote the full sequence of monocyte activation [120]. Elevated levels of plasma lipoproteins, especially low- and very low density frac-tions, may be injurious to the endothelium [54], may permit monocyte adhesion, induce growth factor formation [74], and seem to be linked to arachidonic acid metabolism [46]. Furthermore, it has been demonstrated in cell culture systems that PDGF leads to subsequent activation of the phospholipase C/diglyceride

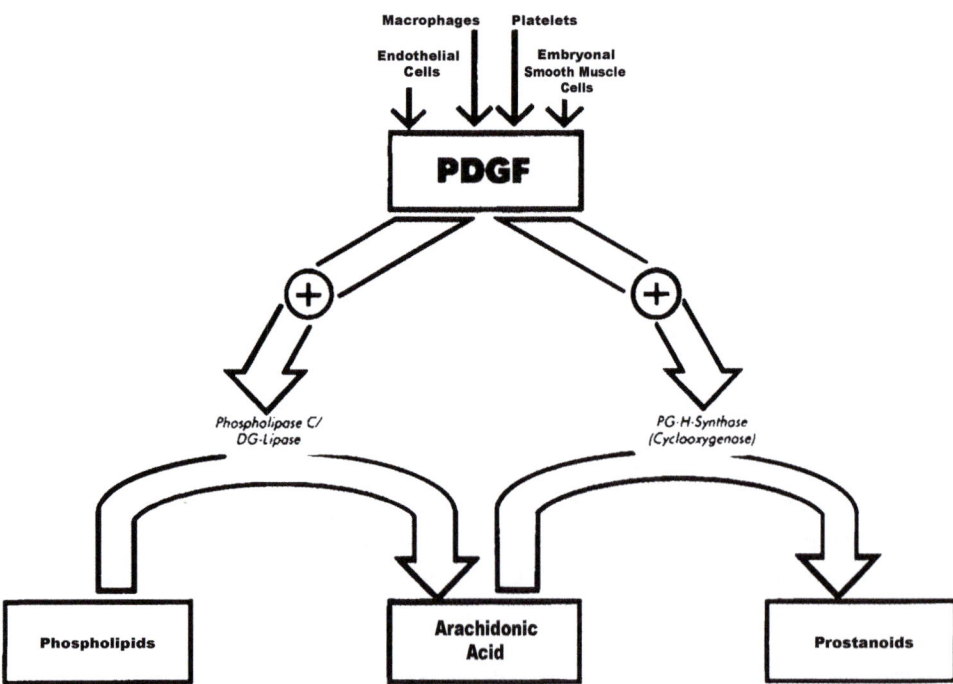

Fig. 1. Platelet-derived growth factor (PDGF) increases phospholipase C/diglyceride lipase-mediated arachidonic acid release, stimulates PGH synthase activity, and induces de novo synthesis of this enzyme

lipase pathway, enhanced release of arachidonic acid, and both activation and de novo synthesis of the key enzyme of prostanoid synthesis, PGH synthase ([44, 45]; Fig. 1).

Clusters of monocytes/macrophages apparently synthesize eicosanoids like thromboxane (TX) A_2 or the peptidoleukotrienes C_4, D_4, and E_4, which promote platelet aggregation and cause vascular constriction [38, 71, 73, 82, 88, 119]; this may explain the reduced blood flow during atherogenesis [74]. Leukocytes produce the potent chemoattractant leukotriene (LT) B_4 [73], which promotes leukocyte migration and the intramural deposition of clusters of white blood cells. Infiltration of myelomonocytic cells or activation of tissue-resident macrophages will potentially increase the locally available amount of eicosanoid synthetic enzymes, implying a probably enhanced cellular vulnerability in case of phospholipase activation and arachidonate release.

Many aspects of atherogenesis are only partially understood. The sequences of hormonally and humorally induced cellular responses, the relative importance of distinct secretory products, and the wide range of genetic features are not well delineated. Only intensive research in the field of the molecular biology of the arterial wall will help to develop a more fundamental understanding of the pathobiology of atherosclerosis [107].

Atherogenesis and Diet

The conclusion that diet and occlusive vascular disease are causally linked is based on the following clinical and experimental observations:

1. Epidemiologic studies have established a close association between the consumption of cholesterol, saturated fat, and total fat, and the incidence of coronary heart disease.
2. Patients with hereditary hyperlipidemia suffer from premature development of coronary heart disease.
3. Serum cholesterol and lipoprotein levels have been shown to be closely correlated not only with variables of fat-modified dietary regimens but also with the occurrence of atherosclerotic lesions which may contain excessive amounts of cholesterol deposits.

The recognition that there is an obvious connection between dietary habits and the so-called coronary epidemic, together with the observation that polyunsaturated fat is able to lower blood cholesterol levels, led to the dietary recommendation of a high daily intake of polyunsaturated fat.

Epidemiologic Data

More than 30 years ago, a marked fall was reported in mortality from cardiovascular disease and in the incidence of myocardial infarction in Norway during

Table 2. Age-adjusted differences in morbidity from chronic diseases between Greenland Eskimos and Danes (modified from Kromann and Green, Acta Med. Scand 208:401, 1980)

	Incidence (Eskimos/Danes)
Myocardial infarction	1:10
Stroke	2:1
Psoriasis	1:20
Bronchial asthma	1:25
Malignant disorders	1:1

the Second World War, obviously due to dietary changes caused by food shortages and associated with a substantial increase in fish consumption.

Descriptive epidemiologic studies comparing Greenland Eskimos and mainland Danes suggested that a diet rich in marine lipids may lead to a significant reduction in the incidence of occlusive vascular disease (Table 2) independent of sex differences and independent of the total amount of fat consumed [7, 8, 26, 87]. The average individual fish consumption of adult Eskimos following traditional dietary habits is estimated to be about 400 g/day [5, 6], i.e., four to six times more than that of mainland Danes.

Low death rates from coronary heart disease were also reported from Japan [57], where the average per capita fish consumption is also traditionally high and is estimated to be about 100 g/day [55]. Within Japan, the island of Okinawa has the lowest incidence of coronary heart disease and a fish consumption which largely exceeds those of the other Japanese regions [55]. Another Japanese study revealed that in a fishing village where the average fish consumption amounted to about 300 g/day, the mortality from coronary heart disease was significantly lower than that of a farming village where the average fish consumption was less than 90 g/day [52].

It is interesting that hand in hand with Westernized dietary habits, disease patterns have changed in Japan and in Greenland and are now characterized by a tendency toward an increased number of deaths from coronary heart disease. Studies based on dietary history have suggested that even a small intake of fish may be able to reduce the incidence of coronary heart disease [60, 108]. An inverse dose-response relation was observed between fish consumption and death from coronary heart disease during 20 years of follow-up in a Dutch population of more than 850 middle-aged men [60]. To compare the relative risk as a function of the amount of fish consumed, individuals who ate no fish at all were assigned a risk level of 1.0. The risk ratios of those consuming 1–14 g, 15–29 g, or 30–144 g of fish were 0.64, 0.56, and 0.36, respectively. The authors of this study concluded that the consumption of as little as one or two fish meals per week may be of preventive value for coronary heart disease [60].

Dietary and Metabolic Data

The most remarkable dietary difference between Arctic or Japanese and European or North American populations has clearly been demonstrated to be the composition of ingested polyunsaturated fatty acids. The primary polyunsaturated fatty acids in the Eskimo or Japanese diet are of the ω-3 family, consisting largely of eicosapentaenoic acid (20:5, ω-3) and docosahexaenoic cid (22:6, ω-3) rather than linoleic acid (18:2, ω-6), which is the predominant polyunsaturated fatty acid in the so-called average or Western diet ([6, 99]; Table 3).

Polyunsaturated fatty acids are ultimately derived from plants, seed, leaves, and phytoplankton. Terrestrial food chains (i.e., edible plants and animal fat) contain primarily linoleic acid (Table 3, Fig. 2), an ω-6 polyunsaturated fatty acid, and only very small amounts of ω-3 polyunsaturated fatty acids (nearly exclusively α-linolenic acid). Fatty acids in land plants are not chain-elongated above the 18-carbon level. In mammalians, the polyunsaturated 18-carbon ω-6 linoleic acid will be converted to arachidonic acid (20:4, ω-6) by chain elongation and desaturation. As the three major families of unsaturated fatty acids (oleic acid, ω-9; linoleic acid, ω-6; and linolenic acid, ω-3) (Table 3) are metabolically nearly inconvertible in mammalians, phytoplankton and algae, which synthesize eicosapentaenoic acid (20:5, ω-3) and docosahexaenoic acid (22:6, ω-3), are the principal sources of the major ω-3 fatty acids. Only α-linolenic acid from vegetable oils is in principle able to be partially converted to eicosapentaenoic acid ([26]; Fig. 2).

All forms of life depending on the marine food chain potentially become enriched with ω-3 fatty acids, and fish may contain extraordinarily high amounts

Table 3. Nomenclature, structure, and dietary sources of the major polyunsaturated fatty acids

Nomenclature			Dietary sources
Family	Fatty acid	Structure	
ω-3	Eicosapentaenoic acid (20:5, ω-3)	H_3C ∿∿ $^{R\,COOH}$ ₃	Fish oils
ω-6	Linoleic acid (18:2, ω-6)	H_3C ∿∿∿ ^{6} $^{R\,COOH}$	Vegetable oils
ω-9	Oleic acid (18:1, ω-9)	H_3C ∿∿∿∿ $^{R\,COOH}$	Vegetable oils, animal fats

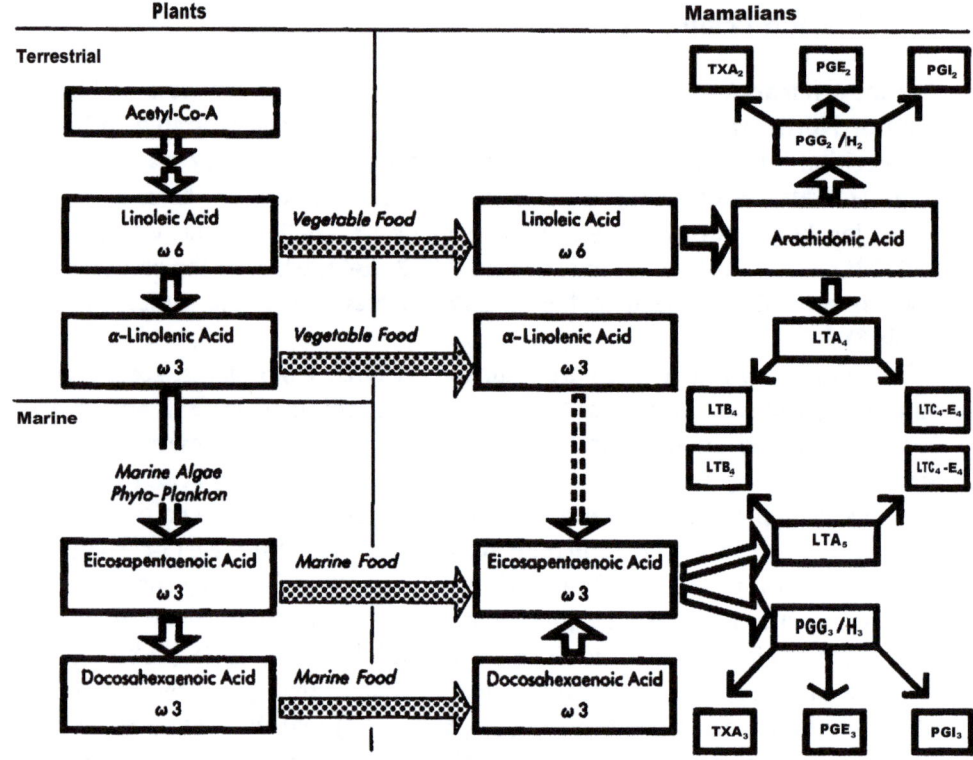

Fig. 2. Origin and metabolism of polyunsaturated ω-6 and ω-3 fatty acids

of eicosapentaenoic or docosahexaenoic acid (Fig. 2). Our present knowledge of the incorporation of dietary ω-6 and ω-3 polyunsaturated fatty acids into organ lipids suggests that, in contrast to the 18-carbon ω-6 polyunsaturated fatty acids, the 20- and 22-carbon ω-3 polyunsaturated fatty acids have to be supplied as such to increase the body stores of these particular acids significantly. In humans, docosahexaenoic acid can be retroconveted to eicosapentaenoic acid [32, 103] and may serve as an additional source of the latter.

A relative selectivity in the incorporation of eicosapentaenoic acid and docosahexaenoic acid into membrane phospholipid pools of platelets and white blood cells has been demonstrated. After 6 days to 4 weeks of fish oil supplementation, a marked increase in the relative eicosapentaenoic acid content of phosphatidylcholine and phosphatidylethanolamine was noted, whereas either no or a relatively minor incorporation in phosphatidylserine and posphatidylinositol could be detected [1, 35, 77, 103, 113]. These results support the hypothesis that the phospholipid acid composition may possibly de determined to a considerable extent during the formative stage of white blood cells, and there is some evidence that these cells do not incorporate eicosapentaenoic acid from the surrounding milieu [103]. Furthermore, the ω-6 fatty acids appear to be favored in the competition for the same enzyem systems metabolizing both ω-6 and ω-3 fatty acids. That means that a relatively high amount of incorporated ω-3 fatty acids would be necessary to reduce arachidonic acid metabolism.

In summary, because humans are not able to convert ω-3 to ω-6 polyunsaturated fatty acids, administration of diets enriched with ω-3 polyunsaturated fatty acids represents the principal and unique possibility of influencing metabolic mechanisms of clinical and therapeutic importance by substrate exchange.

Two aspects of dietary studies deserve considerable attention. First, fish oil is a heterogeneous mixture of fatty acids, with ω-3 fatty acids, i.e., eicosapentaenoic and docosahexaenoic acid, being prevalent in fish flesh with a range of 0.1% – 90% by weight among different species of seafood [74]. Among fish in the Western diet, only mackerel, salmon, albacore tuna, oyster, anchovy, halibut, and herring are rich in ω-3 fatty acids, suggesting a very differentiated view of potential dietary recommendations. Second, we have to point out that eicosapentaenoic acid was administered in some studies in different chemical forms. For example, esterified polyunsaturated fatty acids exhibit a greater metabolic stability than the respective free fatty acids. Furthermore, different chemical forms of eicosapentaenoic acid exhibit striking differences in intraluminal hydrolysis and subsequent intestinal absorption [14]. Therefore, it is possible that different pharmacodynamic properties may have influenced the results of some studies.

Clinical Aspects of Dietary Studies

In most animal models, the course of experimentally induced vascular occlusive disease is independent of risk factors such as smoking, diabetes, or hypertension; this is not the case in humans. Animal experiments are only rough indications of human conditions, and the postulated protective mechanisms of ω-3 polyunsaturated fatty acids may differ substantially from those in humans. Therefore, results of animal studies are obviously not directly applicable to pathophysiologic or therapeutic concepts in human disease.

However, it has been shown that both coronary artery disease and the platelet and coagulation systems in swine are very similar to those in humans, and that the clinical syndromes of sudden death and acute myocardial infarction appear to be comparable [63, 64, 122]. Recently, it was demonstrated that after dietary supplementation with cod-liver oil severely hyperlipidemic swine exhibit retarded atherosclerotic disease development, with no relation to changes in plasma lipids, but associated with changes in the arachidonate and eicosapentaenoic acid content of platelet membranes [123]. Moreover, cats fed with menhaden oil showed significantly smaller neurological deficits after ligation of the left middle cerebral artery [13], and dogs fed with cod-liver oil exhibited smaller sizes of infarcted myocardial tissue than controls after electrical stimulation of the left circumflex coronary artery [22].

Few studies are available to evaluate the clinical benefit of administration of eicosapentaenoic acid. A total of 107 patients with angina pectoris consumed

1.8 – 3.6 g eicosapentaenoic acid and were followed up for 2 years. A decline in nitroglycerin medication from almost 30 to approx. 5 tablets per week has been observed, but no objective data to quantitate the reduction in myocardial ischemia have been reported [101]. Changes in serum lipids, bleeding time, eicosanoid production, platelet aggregation, and neutrophil count after eicosapentaenoic acid or fish-oil-supplemented diets have been demonstrated, but no data were provided about the clinical course of symptoms of occlusive vascular disease [50, 59]; nor could changes in angina frequency and nitroglycerin consumption be observed [74]. The short duration of these studies (5 – 13 weeks) might explain the absence of clinically beneficial effects. Only in one study [74] did decreased blood pressure and heart rate at rest and during exercise indirectly indicate a reduction in myocardial oxygen demand after eicosapentaenoic acid administration.

Biologic Effects on Plasma Lipids

Over the past 25 years, many studies revealed that large amounts of polyunsaturated fat in the daily diet have pronounced hypolipidemic effects [42, 94]. The investigations have largely been focused on the effects of vegetable oils, such as corn and safflower oil, containing large amounts of linoleic acid (18:2, ω-6). The addition of polyunsaturated fat to a fat-free diet resulted in a reduction of plasma cholesterol. The possibility that hypercholesterolemia was induced by essential fatty acid deficiency was discounted when plasma cholesterol levels were effectively reduced by fish oil containing high amounts of ω-3 polyunsaturated fatty acids and only low amounts of linoleic acid [2] (Table 4). Eskimos following their traditional life-style have lower blood levels of very low density lipoprotein

Table 4. Biologic effects of ω-3 polyunsaturated fatty acids on blood lipids, sterol excretion, and lipogenesis

Parameter	Effect
VLDL cholesterol[a]	↓↓
LDL cholesterol[a]	↓(?)
HDL cholesterol[a]	↑
Total cholesterol[a]	↓(?)
VLDL synthesis rate	↓
Triglycerides[a]	↓↓
Fecal sterol output	↑
Hepatic lipogenesis	↓

[a] Blood.

(VLDL) and higher levels of high-density lipoprotein (HDL) cholesterol, whereas low-density lipoprotein (LDL) levels are not significantly different when compared with the corresponding levels in Eskimos preferring a Western diet [9]. A variety of human and animal studies have shown that fish oils or fish diets reduce VLDL cholesterol [23, 29, 70, 89], whereas LDL cholesterol concentrations are only decreased when large amounts of ω-3 polyunsaturated fatty acids (90 – 120 g daily) are ingested [53]. Other studies have demonstrated that ω-3 polyunsaturated fatty acids are approximately as hypocholesterolemic as polyunsaturated vegetable oils [39, 41, 49]. Controlled feeding experiments have shown that dietary ω-3 fatty acids did not change or even increased concentrations of HDL [17, 23, 70, 89, 98]. Moreover, a large British group of regular daily fish eaters had significantly higher HDL cholesterol levels than meat eaters or vegetarians [118].

Two interesting features of these studies deserve special comments. First, since fish oils contain large amounts of cholesterol (300 – 500 mg/dl) [51] and vegetable oils contain none, the finding that similar hypocholesterolemic effects are produced by these two types of fat implies that fish oils might have been even more hypocholesterolemic if they had not contained dietary cholesterol [124]. Therefore, variations in the lipid load could partially explain some conflicting data to the effect that administration of relatively moderate doses of fish oils did not clearly reveal hypocholesterolemic effects or has even been observed to increase blood cholesterol levels [24]. This view is supported by results indicating that only large amounts of fish oil will be able to inhibit the rise in blood cholesterol usually seen in association with the unavoidable simultaneous ingestion of cholesterol [84]. Second, the daily intake of ω-6 fatty acids was invariably greater than the intake of ω-3 fatty acids, a fact which has to be kept in mind when the lipid-lowering effects of ω-6 and ω-3 polyunsaturated fatty acids are compared.

Furthermore, considerable reduction in the concentration of plasma triglycerides and a significant decrease in the VLDL production rate [83] have been observed in both normolipidemic and hyperlipidemic subjects after dietary fish oil supplementation [41]. This lipid-lowering effect has been shown to be directly proportional to the pretreatment serum triglyceride levels [89]. Direct comparison of the effects of fish and vegetable oils revealed that blood triglyceride levels fell only as a result of the fish diets, suggesting that fish oils possess unique hypotriglyceridemic properties not found in the polyunsaturated ω-6 fatty acids or vegetable oils [41].

Significant lipid-lowering effects usually occur within 2 – 4 weeks after the onset of the fish oil diet, and further decreases may be observed up to 2 years later [59, 89, 101]. The pathophysiological mechanisms of the lipid-lowering effects are not known. There is only some evidence that ω-3 (as well as ω-6) fatty acids stimulate the fecal output of neutral and acidic sterols [41] and may inhibit hepatic lipogenesis [125] (Table 4).

Data on Fatty Acid Composition of Adipose Tissue

The Edinburgh-Stockholm study demonstrated a significantly lower proportion of linoleic acid in adipose tissue of healthy men in Edinburgh than in a comparable group in Stockholm; this was associated with a coronary heart disease mortality which was three times higher in Edinburgh [68]. Cross-cultural and cross-sectional surveys indicated that people in areas with high coronary heart disease mortality have low levels of linoleic acid in adipose tissue [93, 126]. Recently, inverse relations were reported between the content of linoleic acid in adipose tissue and of eicosapentaenoic acid in platelet membranes and the estimated relative risk of angina pectoris and acute myocardial infarction [127]. Hardly any eicosapentaenoic acid is present in adipose tissue in Western populations [28]. Even after 74 days of a diet enriched with eicosapentaenoic acid (14 g daily) only 0.5% of eicosapentaenoic acid was incorporated into adipose tissue [111]. In contrast, ingestion of a fish oil diet significantly decreased the content of linoleic acid in adipose tissue [111]. These changes in the fatty acid composition of adipose tissue appear to depend not only on the pattern and the amount of fatty acids in the various diets but also on that of carbohydrates and on the amount of adipose tissue. There is evidence that low intake of linoleic acid or a low content of linoleic acid in serum phospholipids may also predispose to myocardial infarction [75, 110], indicating complex and univestigated biologic mechanisms and interactions between eicosapentaenoic acid and linoleic acid.

Biologic Effects on Eicosanoid Synthesis

Arachidonic acid (20:4, ω-6), derived directly from dietary sources as well as from the conversion of linoleic acid (18:2, ω-6), is a major component of membrane phospholipids and the principal substrate for prostanoid and leukotriene synthesis in mammalians ([37], Fig. 3). Arachidonic acid is converted in platelets through the PGH synthase (cyclooxygenase) pathway to products with two double bonds (such as thromboxane A_2, a potent vasoconstrictor and platelet aggregatory agent) and in the endothelium of blood vessels to prostacyclin, a potent vasodilator and platelet inhibitor (Table 5). Excessive thromboxane release has been implicated in the genesis and propagation of atherosclerosis and myocardial ischemia, resulting in unstable angina pectoris and acute myocardial infarction [72, 86]. In leukocytes, arachidonic acid is converted along the lipoxygenase pathway to leukotrienes (LT) of the 4-series and hydroxy fatty acids. LTA_4 is an unstable epoxide derivative of arachidonic acid. It is hydrolated enzymatically to LTB_4, which causes an increase in vascular permeability and enhanced chemotaxis of white blood cells. A second metabolic pathway leads [after the conjugation of LTA_4 with glutathione (LTC_4) and the successive elimination of a γ-glutamyl residue (LTD_4) and of glycine (LTE_4)] to the peptidoleukotrienes C_4, D_4, and E_4, which cause coronary artery constriction and platelet activation ([37, 73, 121]; Table 5).

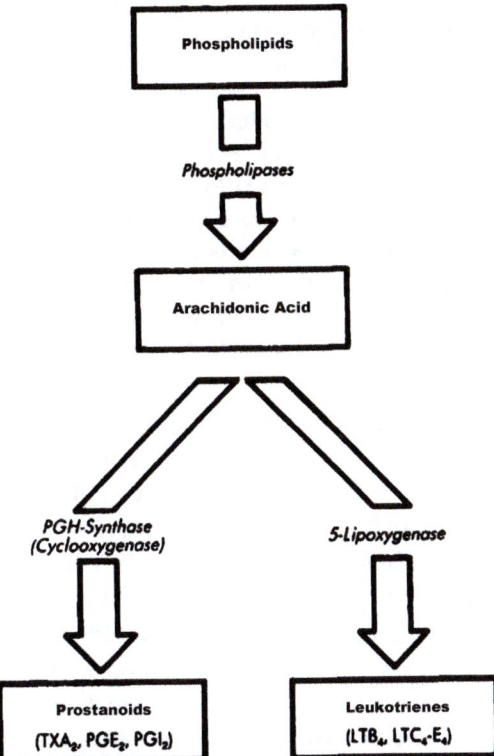

Fig. 3. Arachidonic acid is metabolized either by the PGH synthase/cyclooxygenase enzymatic system or by 5-lipoxygenases to metabolically active prostanoids or leukotrienes (or will be reacetylated into membrane-bound phospholipids)

Table 5. Comparison of biologic properties of eicosanoids synthesized from arachidonic acid (AA; 20:4, ω-6) or eicosapentaenoic acid (EPA; 20:5, ω-3)

Cellular origin	AA	EPA
Platelets	Thromboxane A_2: Vasoconstriction Platelet Aggregation	Thromboxane A_3: No or weak vaso- constriction or aggregation
Endothelium	Prostaglandin I_2: Vasodilation Antiaggregation	Prostaglandin I_3: Vasodilation Antiaggregation
Neutrophils/monocytes	Leukotriene B_4: Strong chemotaxis Leukotriene C_4: Vasoconstriction Bronchoconstriction	Leukotriene B_5: Weak chemotaxis Leukotriene C_5: Inactive

Table 6. Biologic effects of ω-3 polyunsaturated fatty acids on eicosanoid synthesis

---

Decrease of phospholipase activity
Poor substrate for the PGH synthase
Preferential substrate(s) for the 5-lipoxygenase
Thromboxane A_3 is less potent than thromboxane A_2
Prostaglandin I_3 activity is similar to that of prostaglandin I_2
Leukotrienes of the 5-series are less potent than those of the 4-series
Leukotriene A_5 inhibits leukotriene A_4 formation

Eicosapentaenoic acid (Table 6) is easily incorporated into the cell membrane-bound phospholipids. It is a poor substrate for the cyclooxygenase/hydroperoxidase enzymatic system, and only very small amounts of endproducts with three double bonds will be formed when compared with the relative effectiveness of arachidonate metabolism. In contrast, eicosapentaenoic acid is a preferred substrate for product generation by the 5-lipoxygenase in subcellular fractions of human and animal neutrophils [66, 87], whereas docosahexaenoic acid is also a markedly inferior substrate for leukotriene synthesis. Eicosapentaenoic acid appears to inhibit phospholipase activity, resulting in a decrease of arachidonic acid release ([67]; Fig. 4). Moreover, simultaneously with thromboxane A_3 and prostaglandin I_3 generation from eicosapentaenoic acid, the synthesis of thromboxane A_2 and prostacyclin (PGI_2) from arachidonic acid [47] decreases, mainly due to inhibitory effects on PGH synthase activity (Fig. 4).

Thromboxane A_3 is considerably less potent than its counterpart thromboxane A_2, whereas prostaglandin I_3 exhibits biologic activities which appear to be similar to those of the arachidonate-derived prostacyclin (PGI_2) (Table 5). Indeed, recently it has been shown that the balance between prostacyclin and thromboxane is shifted in favor of prostacyclin synthase products in Greenland Eskimos as compared with the Danish control population [31]. Because eicosapentaenoic acid is a preferential substrate for the 5-lipoxygenase, subsequent formation of leukotrienes of the 5-series (which are much less potent than those of the 4-series) will be favored by administration of ω-3 polyunsaturated fatty acids [65, 90, 116]. Furthermore, LTA_5 leads to a substantial decrease in the formation of LTA_4 by direct inhibitory effects on the LT hydrolase system ([80]; Fig. 4). The available data indicate that at least in neutrophils the pattern of formed leukotrienes is substantially changed in favour of a relative decrease of LTB_4 synthesis by dietary eicosapentaenoic acid administration.

Docosahexaenoic acid is not a substrate for the prostaglandin synthetic system but is capable of competitive inhibition of the PGH synthase (cyclooxygenase) activity from ram seminal vesicles ([20]; Fig. 4) without significant interference with the conversion of arachidonic acid to leukotrienes [20]. The docosahexaenoic acid which is not metabolized to eicosapentaenoic acid will be oxygenated to inactive substances at least by human platelets [4].

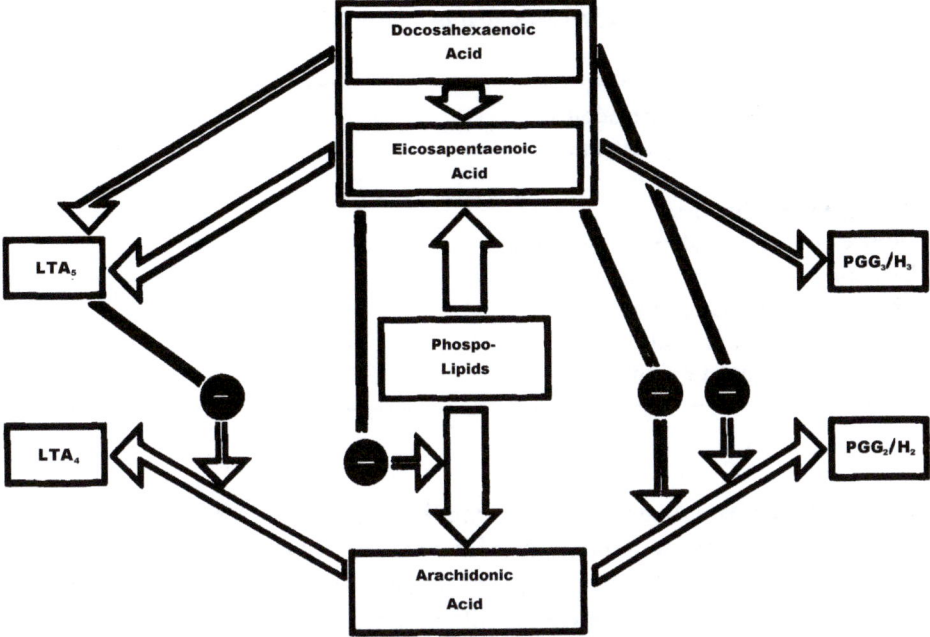

Fig. 4. Inhibitory effects of eicosapentaenoic acid and its metabolites on arachidonic acid metabolism which have been shown in in vitro systems

In summary, eicosapentaenoic and docosahexaenoic acid competitively inhibit the utilization of arachidonic acid by the PGH synthase [25, 81] and consequently decrease the available amount of metabolites of arachidonic acid, thus promoting the synthesis of biologically less active eicosanoids from eicosapentaenoic acid [29, 67, 81, 113].

Biologic Effects on Platelets, Hemostasis, and Blood Viscosity

Platelet abnormalities indicating platelet hyperreactivity have been identified in patients with myocardial ischemia [72]. The coagulation cascade is activated at sites of atherosclerotic plaque rupture, where platelet adhesion to exposed subendothelial collagen and microfibrils may occur. Dietary studies on normal human volunteers have shown that the supplementation of Western diet with sea fish or fish oil containing high amounts of eicosapentaenoic and docosahexaenoic acid induces a significant reduction of platelet aggregation, associated with a prolonged bleeding time ([15, 97, 104, 109]; Table 7). Even 10 ml eicosapentaenoic acid per day or 500−800 g mackerel per day for 2−3 weeks exhibits these potentially beneficial effects, paralleled by an increase in the content of incorporated eicosapentaenoic and docosahexaenoic acid and a significant reduction in the amount of cellular-bound ω-6 polyunsaturated fatty acids in platelet and red-cell membranes [1, 40, 59, 69, 109]. These findings are con-

Table 7. Biologic effects of polyunsaturated ω-3 fatty acids on platelets, hemostasis, and blood viscosity

---

Reduction of platelet aggregation
Altered distribution of platelet size
Reduction of platelet count
Prolonged bleeding time
Decrease of thromboxane A_2 generation
Decrease of β-thromboglobulin synthesis
Changes in erythrocyte fluidity
Decrease of blood viscosity
Increase of fibrinolytic activity

---

sistent with epidemiologic data indicating that a prolonged bleeding time and low platelet counts occur in populations with a very high intake of fish oil [59]. More modest ingestion of fish (200 g/day) or fish oil (20 g/day) prolongs bleeding time without any reduction of platelet counts or clotting factors [69, 98].

Associated with the decline in platelet aggregation and the increased bleeding time, severely decreased thromboxane A_2 generation and additional prolongation of the bleeding time after aspirin administration have been documented [1, 50, 109, 117]. High doses of eicosapentaenoic acid (10 g/day) given for 1 month have been shown to effectively alter the pattern of prostanoid synthesis [59], however, platelet functions were only moderately reduced in some studies, consistent with an incomplete suppression of thromboxane A_2 synthesis [40, 59]. A residual capacity of only about 10% to synthesize thromboxane A_2 has been shown to be sufficient to sustain platelet aggregation [27]. In addition, the relation between inhibition of thromboxane A_2 formation and thromboxane-dependent platelet functions has been found not to be linear [62]. Dose-related effects on platelet aggregation have been clearly demonstrated in healthy volunteers after ingestion of cod-liver oil or eicosapentaenoic acid [62, 79, 102, 115]. Prostacyclin (PGI_2) biosynthesis appears to be unchanged during the formation of prostaglandin I_3 in healthy humans placed on a diet rich in fish oils [29], whereas the increased prostacyclin synthesis of atherosclerotic patients seems to be markedly reduced after only 1 week [59]. The prolongation of the bleeding time, reduction of β-thromboglobulin levels, and shift in the distribution of platelets according to size have been described as only moderate effects after eicosapentaenoic acid administration, but they are nevertheless potentially important in a complex system of cellular and hormonal interactions.

Docosahexaenoic acid not only is able to be retroconverted to eicosapentaenoic acid but also seems to directly reduce platelet responsiveness [92, 103], as well as platelet PGH synthase activity [20]. There is good evidence for the assumption that eicosapentaenoic acid and docosahexaenoic acid affect platelet aggregation via different mechanisms [4, 30, 103]. In addition to the inhibitory effects on endogenous arachidonic acid metabolism, when preloaded into the membrane-bound phospholipids, docosahexaenoic acid seems to act directly on the membrane level to reduce platelet aggregation [21].

Dietary supplements of polyunsaturated ω-3 fatty acids induce changes in membrane-associated cell functions and membrane physical properties such as fluidity [56, 58, 114]. Eicosapentaenoic acid strongly decreases blood viscosity relative to alterations of the phospholipid content in red blood cell membranes [19, 128]. Furthermore, an enhancing effect of ω-3 fatty acids on plasma fibrinolysis has been reported [10; Table 7].

Biologic Effects on White Blood Cells and Inflammation

White blood cells play a central role in tissue damage. Tissue injury triggers an inflammatory-type reaction, with subsequent infiltration of neutrophils and monocytes and activation of tissue-resident macrophages. The invading cells are able to synthesize and release a variety of proinflammatory mediators, which exacerbate the damage produced by the initial injurious stimulus. These biologically potent mediators cause platelet activation and vasoconstriction, increase vascular permeability, and strongly enhance neutrophil and monocyte migration. Abnormalities of platelet and leukocyte responsiveness are important factors that potentially determine the process of thrombus formation and may even be responsible for the propagation of the atherosclerotic process itself. Increased neutrophil aggregation in patients with acute myocardial infarction [12] and accumulation of mast cells in the coronary arteries of patients with vasospastic angina [34] may contribute to myocardial ischemia by release of histamine, prostanoids, and leukotrienes. Infiltration of leukocytes into so-called platelet clots is considered to partially determine arterial thrombus formation in narrowed coronary arteries, while neutrophil invasion appears to critically determine the size of myocardial infarction [11, 78, 95, 105].

Studies of myocardial ischemia, pulmonary embolism, and endotoxin-induced injury have shown that agents which prevent activation and infiltration of leukocytes reduce the extent of local tissue damage [76]. A decrease in the number of leukocytes by use of antineutrophil serum or inhibition of leukocyte function by pharmacologic agents not only decreases the extent of platelet deposition in ischemic myocardium but also reduces intracoronary thrombus formation and the size of the infarcted area in animal models of myocardial ischemia [11, 78, 95, 105].

Dietary enrichment with eicosapentaenoic (3.2 g/day) and docosahexaenoic (2.2 g/day) acid for only 6 weeks resulted in a significant alteration in membrane composition [91] and cellular functions of monocytes and neutrophils, which reverted to pretreatment values about 6 weeks after stopping supplementation [67] (Table 8). The eicosapentaenoic acid content of cell membranes of white blood cells increased without altering the amount of membrane-bound arachi-

Table 8. Biologic effects of polyunsaturated ω-3 fatty acids on white blood cells and inflammatory reactions

---

Reduction of eicosanoid synthesis of monocytes and neutrophils
Decrease of neutrophil chemotaxis
Impairment of neutrophil endothelial adherence
Decreased neutrophil phagocytosis
Decreased myelomonocytic superoxide production

---

donic acid. However, the release of the substrate arachidonic acid and the biosynthesis of prostanoids of the 2-series and of leukotrienes of the 4-series were dramatically reduced [67, 91]. Furthermore, neutrophil chemotaxis and endothelial adherence were also significantly reduced 6 weeks after the onset of the supplemented diet [67]. After 6 weeks of daily cod-liver oil ingestion, phagocytosing polymorphonuclear leukocytes demonstrated a nearly 64% decrease in superoxide production [33].

The complex interactions between the vascular endothelium and the blood leukocytes are of major interest [48]. One aspect is that neutrophils as well as monocytes and macrophages promote endothelial injury through the release of potentially cytotoxic free oxygen radicals, which partially seem to be generated along the PGH synthase and lipoxygenase pathways [61]. The initial response of neutrophils and probably monocytes to an inflammatory focus appears to be attenuated by the impaired endothelical-cell adherence after eicosapentaenoic acid administration. Furthermore, the decrease in production of LTB_4, the most active natural chemotactic factor [18, 112], would additionally diminish the amplifying functions of neutrophils and monocytes.

In summary, the net result of a diet enriched with fish-oil-derived fatty acids in a potentially inflammatory process appears to be a decrease in the eicosanoid synthesis of myelomonocytic cells, with preferential inhibition of the formation of leukotrienes of the 4-series and a parallel loss of functional competence of these inflammatory cells.

Future Considerations

The effects of ω-3 polyunsaturated fatty acids on platelet, neutrophil, and monocyte functions, membrane fluidity, serum lipids, and both prostanoid and leukotriene formation are aspects of a fundamental modulation of complex interactions between different cellular systems [16] and may be potentially important in the pathobiology of atherosclerosis [36, 106, 107]. Moreover, recent investigations indicated that other substances in addition to ω-3 polyunsaturated fatty acids may be responsible for the antithrombotic properties of marine fish [3], a point which has to be evaluated in the future.

But in spite of the potential usefulness of ω-3 fatty acids in the treatment of occlusive vascular disease, it has to be pointed out that a balanced view of any new form of therapy is absolutely essential. There are too many questions remaining, and consequently we must not be overenthusiastic. Animal experiments are only rough indications of human conditions, and the metabolism and transport mechanisms for polyunsaturated fatty acids may differ substantially from those in humans.

Very few studies (which cannot easily be compared with one another) are available to evaluate the clinical benefit of dietary ω-3 polyunsaturated fatty acids. There are conflicting data concerning the effects of eicosapentaenoic acid on hypercholesterolemia and the relevance of the accompanying lipid load. Furthermore, prostacyclin does not only have antiaggregatory effects; there is some evidence that prostacyclin may be able to increse the hydrolysis of cholesterol esters, at least in arterial smooth muscle cells. Moreover, the following point needs to be kept in mind: it has been reported not only that Eskimos have a lower incidence of occlusive vascular disease than their Danish counterparts but also that the incidence of stroke in Eskimos is about twofold (Table 2), and that their longevity is not higher. The safety of long-term ingestion of high doses of fish oils remains to be sufficiently established [85]. In fact, myocardial fibrosis and lipidosis have been observed in animal experiments after prolonged administration of large quantities of fish oil (100). We have to consider that large doses of fish oil should be regarded as pharmacologic agents which have to meet the appropriate medical requirements rather than as nutritional supplements. Furthermore, the degree of changes in platelet functions even 1 month after daily ingestion of high doses of fish oil is much smaller than 1 h after a single aspirin tablet [59].

Only controlled clinical trials and intervention trials with mortality or defined clinical events as end points (rather than biochemical or in vitro studies) are able to sufficiently test the effectiveness of ω-3 fatty acids in human disease and may potentially provide a basis for recommendations on dietary ω-3 supplementation in humans.

References

1. Ahmed AA, Holub BJ (1984) Alterations and recovery of bleeding times, platelet aggregation, and fatty acid composition of individual phospholipids in platelets of human subjects receiving a supplement of cod liver oil. Lipids 19:617–624
2. Ahrens EH, Insull W, Hirsch J (1959) The effect on human serum lipids of dietary fat, highly unsaturated but poor in essential fatty acids. Lancet 1:115–119
3. Atkinson PM, Wheeler MC, Mendelsohn D, Pienaar N, Chetty N (1987) Effects of a 4-week freshwater fish (trout) diet on platelet aggregation, platelet fatty acids, serum lipids, and coagulation factors. Am J Hematol 24:143–149
4. Aveldano MI, Sprecher H (1983) Synthesis of hydroxy fatty acids from 4,7,10,13,16,19-/1-14C) docosahexaenoic acid by human platelets. J Biol Chem 258:9339–9343

5. Bang HO, Dyerberg J (1972) Plasma lipids and lipoproteins in Greenlandic west coast Eskimos. Acta Med Scand 192:85–94

6. Bang HO, Dyerberg J, Hjorne N (1976) The composition of food consumed by Greenland Eskimos. Acta Med Scand 200:69–73

7. Bang HO, Dyerberg J, Sinclair HM (1980) The composition of the Eskimo food in north western Greenland. Am J Clin Nutr 33:2657–2661

8. Bang HO, Dyerberg J (1980) The bleeding tendency in Greenland Eskimos. Dan Med Bull 27:202–205

9. Bang HO, Dyerberg J (1980) The lipid metabolism and ischemic heart disease in Greenland Eskimos. Adv Nutr Res 3:1–8

10. Barcelli U, Glas-Greenwalt P, Pollak VE (1985) Enhancing effect of dietary supplementation with omega-3 fatty acids on plasma fibrinolysis in normal subjects. Thromb Res 39:307–312

11. Bednar M, Smith B, Pinto A, Mullane KM (1985) Neutrophil depletion suppresses In-labeled platelet accumulation in infarcted myocardium. J Cardiovasc Pharmacol 7:906–912

12. Berliner S, Sclarovski S, Lavie G, Pinkhas J, Aronson M, Agmon J (1986) The leukergy test in patients with ischemic heart disease. Am Heart J 111:19–22

13. Black KL, Culp B, Madison D, Randell OS, Lands WEM (1979) The protective effects of dietary fish oil on focal cerebral infarction. Prostaglandins Med 3:257–268

14. Boustani SEl, Colette C, Monnier L, Descomps B, Crastes de Paulet A, Mendy F (1987) Enteral absorption in man of eicosapentaenoic acid in different chemical forms. Lipids 22:711–714

15. Bradlow BA, Chetty N, Van der Westhuyzen J, Mendelsohn D, Gibson JE (1983) The effects of a mixed fish diet on platelet function, fatty acids and serum lipids. Thromb Res 29:561–568

16. Bradlow BA (1986) Thrombosis and omega-3 fatty acids: Epidemiological and clinical aspects. In: Simopoulos AP, Kifer RR, Martin RE (eds) Health effects of polyunsaturated fatty acids in sea food. Academic, Orlando

17. Bronsgeest-Schoute HC, van Gent CM, Luten JB, Ruiter A (1981) The effects of various intakes of omega-3 fatty acids on the blood lipid composition in healthy human subjects. Am J Clin Nutr 34:1752–1757

18. Camp RDR, Coutts AA, Greaves MW, Kay AB, Walport JM (1983) Response of human skin to intradermal injection of leukotriene C4, D4, and B4. Br J Pharmacol 80:497–502

19. Cartwright IJ, Pockley AG, Galloway JH, Greaves M, Preston FE (1985) The effects of dietary omega-3 polyunsaturated fatty acids on erythrocyte membrane phospholipids, erythrocyte deformability, and blood viscosity in healthy volunteers. Atherosclerosis 55:267–281

20. Corey EJ, Shih C, Cashman JR (1983) Docosahexaenoic acid is a strong inhibitor of prostaglandin but not leukotriene biosynthesis. Proc Natl Acad Sci USA 80:3581–3584

21. Croset M, Lagarde M (1986) In vitro incorporation and metabolism of icosapentaenoic and docosahexaenoic acids in human platelets – effect on aggregation. Thromb Hemost 56:57–62

22. Culp BR, Lands WEM, Lucchesi BR, Pitt B, Romson J (1980) The effect of dietary supplementation of fish oil on experimental myocardial infarction. Prostaglandins 20:1021–1029

23. Davidson MH, Liebson PR (1986) Marine lipids and atherosclerosis: a review. Cardiovasc Rev Rep 7:461 – 471
24. Demke DM, Peters GR, Linet OI, Metzler CM, Klott KA (1987) The effects of fish oil concentrate, Maxepa, in patients with hypercholesterinemia. 2nd Cardiovascular pharmacotherapy international symposium, Oct 18 – 22, San Francisco
25. Dyerberg J, Bang HO, Stoffersen G, Moncada S, Vane JR (1978) Eicosapentaenoic acid and prevention of thrombosis and atherosclerosis. Lancet 2:117 – 119
26. Dyerberg J (1986) Linolenate-derived polyunsaturated fatty acids and prevention of atherosclerosis. Nutr Rev 44:125 – 134
27. DiMinno G, Silver MG, Murphy S (1983) Monitoring the entry of new platelets into the circulation after ingestion of aspirin. Blood 61:1081 – 1085
28. Field CJ, Angel A, Clandinin MT (1985) Relationship of diet to the fatty acid composition of human adipose tissue structural and stored lipids. Am J Clin Nutr 42:1206 – 1220
29. Fischer S, Weber PC (1984) Prostaglanin I3 is formed in vivo in man after dietary eicosapentaenoic acid. Nature 307:165 – 168
30. Fischer S, von Schacky C, Siess W, Strasser T, Weber PC (1984) Uptake, release, and metabolism of docosahexaenoic acid in human platelets and neutrophils. Biochem Biophys Res Commun 120:907 – 918
31. Fischer S, Weber PC, Dyerberg J (1986) The prostacyclin/thromboxane balance is favourably shifted in Greenland Eskimos. Prostaglandins 32:235 – 241
32. Fischer S, Vischer A, Praec-Mursic, Weber PC (1987) Dietary docosahexaenoic acid is retroconverted in man to eicosapentaenoic acid, which can be quickly transformed to prostaglandin I3. Prostaglandins 34:367 – 375
33. Fisher M, Upchurch KS, Levine PH, Johnson MH, Vaudreuil CH, Natale A, Hoogasian JJ (1986) Effects of dietary fish oil supplementation on polymorphonuclear leukocyte inflammatory potential. Inflammation 10:387 – 392
34. Forman M, Oates JA, Robertson D, Robertson RM, Roberts LJ, Virmani R (1985) Increased adventitial mast cells in a patient with coronary spasm. N Engl J Med 313:1138 – 1141
35. Galloway JH, Cartwright IJ, Woodcock BE, Greaves M, Russell GG, Preston FE (1985) Effects of dietary fish oil supplementation of the fatty acid composition on the human platelet membrane: demonstration of selectivity in the incorporation of eicosapentaenoic acid into membrane phospholipid pools. Clin Sci 68:449 – 454
36. Glomset JA (1985) Fish, fatty acids, and human health. N Engl J Med 312:1253 – 1254
37. Goerig M, Habenicht AJR, Schettler G (1985) Eicosanoide und Phospholipasen. Klin Wochenschrift 63:293 – 311
38. Goerig M, Habenicht AJR, Heitz R, Zeh W, Katus H, Kommerell B, Ziegler R, Glomset JA (1987) Sn-1,2-diacylglycerols and phorbol diesters stimulate thromboxane synthesis by de novo synthesis of prostaglandin H synthase in human promyelocytic leukemia cells. J Clin Invest 79:903 – 911
39. Goldberg AC, Schonfeld G (1985) Effects of diet on lipoprotein metabolism. Ann Rev Nutr 5:195 – 212
40. Goodnight SH, Harris WS, Connor WE (1981) The effects of dietary omega-3 fatty acids on platelet composition and function in man. Blood: 58:880 – 885
41. Goodnight SH, Harris WS, Connor WE, Illingworth DR (1982) Polyunsaturated fatty acids, hyperlipidemia, and thrombosis. Arteriosclerosis 2:87 – 113
42. Grundy SM (1986) Cholesterol and coronary heart disease. A new era. JAMA 256: 2849 – 2858

43. Habenicht AJR, Goerig M, Schettler G (1984) Neue Aspekte der Biochemie und Biologie der Arterienwand. Klin Wochenschrift 62:241–253

44. Habenicht AJR, Glomset JA, Goerig M, Gronwald R, Grulich J, Loth U, Schettler G (1985) Cell cycle-dependent changes in arachidonic acid and glycerol metabolism in Swiss 3T3 cells stimulated by platelet-derived growth factor. J Biol Chem 260:1370–1373

45. Habenicht AJR, Goerig M, Grulich J, Rothe D, Gronwald R, Loth U, Schettler G, Kommerell B, Ross R (1985) Human platelet-derived growth factor stimulates prostaglandin synthesis by activation and by rapid de novo synthesis of cyclooxygenase. J Clin Invest 75:1381–1387

46. Habenicht AJR, Dresel HA, Goerig M, Wever J, Stoehr M, Glomset JA, Ross R, Schettler G (1986) Low density lipoprotein receptor-dependent prostaglandin synthesis in Swiss 3T3 cells stimulated by platelet-derived growth factor. Proc Natl Acad Sci USA 83:1344–1348

47. Hadjiagapiou C, Kaduce TL, Spector AA (1986) Eicosapentaenoic acid utilization by bovine aortic endothelial cells: effects on prostacyclin production. Biochim Biophys Acta 875:369–381

48. Harlan JM (1985) Leukocyte-endothelial interactions. Blood 65:513–525

49. Harris WS, Connor WE (1980) The effects of salmon oil upon plasma lipids, lipoproteins, and triglyceride clearance. Trans Assoc Am Physicians 43:148–155

50. Hay CRM, Durber AP, Saynor R (1982) Effect of fish oil on platelet kinetics in patients with ischaemic heart disease. Lancet 1:1269–1272

51. Hepburn FN, Exler J, Weihrauch JL (1986) Provisional tables on the content of omega-3 fatty acids and other fat components of selected foods. J Am Diet Assoc 86:788–793

52. Hirai A, Hamazaki T, Terano T (1980) Eicosapentaenoic acid and platelet function in Japanese. Lancet 2:1132–1133

53. Illingworth DR, Harris WS, Connor WE (1984) Inhibition of low density lipoprotein synthesis by dietary omega-3 fatty acids in humans. Arteriosclerosis 4:270–275

54. Jackson RL, Gotto AM (1976) Hypothesis concerning membrane structure, cholesterol, and atherosclerosis. In: Paoletti R, Gotto AM Jr (eds) Atherosclerosis reviews, vol 1. Raven, New York, pp 1–21

55. Kagawa Y, Nishizawa M, Suzuki M (1982) Eicosapolyenoic acid of serum lipids of Japanese islanders with low incidence of cardiovascular diseases. J Nutr Sci Vitaminol 28:441–453

56. Kamada T, Yamashita T, Baba Y, Kai M, Setoyama S, Chuman Y, Otsuji S (1986) Dietary sardine oil increases erythrocyte membrane fluidity in diabetic patients. Diabetes 35:604–611

57. Keys A (1980) Seven countries: a multivariate analysis of death and coronary heart disease. Harvard University Press, Cambridge

58. King ME, Stavens BW, Spector AA (1977) Diet-induced changes in plasma membrane fatty acid composition affect physical properties detected with a spin-label probe. Biochemistry 16:5280–5285

59. Knapp HR, Reilly IAG, Allessandrini P, Fitzgerald GA (1986) In vivo indexes of platelet and vascular function during fish-oil administration in patients with atherosclerosis. N Engl J Med 314:937–942

60. Kromhout D, Bosschieter EB, de Lezenne-Coulander C (1985) The inverse relation between fish consumption and 20-year mortality from coronary heart disease. N Engl J Med 312:1205–1209

61. Kukreja RC, Kontos HA, Hess ML, Ellis EF (1986) PGH synthase and lipoxygenase generate superoxide in the presence of NADH or NADPH. Circ Res 59:612–619

62. Lands WEM, Culp BR, Hirai A, Gorman R (1985) Relationship of thromboxane generation to the aggregation of platelets from humans. Effects of eicosapentaenoic acid. Prostaglandins 30:819–825

63. Leach CM, Thorburn GD (1982) A comparative study of collagen induced thromboxane release from platelets of different species: implications for human atherosclerosis models. Prostaglandins 24:47–59

64. Lee KT, Jarmolych J, Kim DN (1971) Production of advanced coronary atherosclerosis, myocardial infarction, and sudden death in swine. Exp Mol Pathol 15:170–190

65. Lee TH, Menica-Huerta JM, Shih C, Corey EJ, Lewis RA, Austen KF (1984) Characterisation and biologic properties of 5,12-dihydroxy derivatives of eicosapentaenoic acid, including leukotriene B5 and the double lipoxygenase product. J Biol Chem 259:2383–2389

66. Lee TH, Menica-Huerta JM, Shih C, Corey EJ, Lewis RA, Austen KF (1984) Effects of exogenous arachidonic, eicosapentaenoic, and docosahexaenoic acids on the generation of 5-lipoxygenase pathway products by ionophore-activated human neutrophils. J Clin Invest 74:1922–1933

67. Lee TE, Hoover RL, Williams JD, Sperling RI, Ravalese J, Spur BW, Robinson DR, Corey EJ, Lewis RA, Austen KF (1985) Effect of dietary enrichment with eicosapentaenoic and docosahexaenoic acids on in vitro neutrophil and monocyte leukotriene generation and neutrophil function. N Engl J Med 312:1217–1224

68. Logan RL, Thomson M, Riemersma RA (1978) Risk factors for ischemic heart disease in normal men aged 40. Lancet i:949–955

69. Lorenz R, Spengler U, Fischer S, Duhm J, Weber PC (1983) Platelet function, thromboxane formation, and blood pressure control during supplementation of the western diet with cod liver oil. Circulation 67:504–511

70. von Lossonczy TO, Ruiter A, Bronsgeest-Schoute HC, van Gent CM, Hermus RJJ (1978) The effect of a fish oil diet on serum lipids in healthy human subjects. Am J Clin Nutr 31:1340–1346

71. Majerus PW (1983) Arachidonate metabolism in vascular disorders. J Clin Invest 72:1521–1525

72. Mehta J (1983) Platelets and prostaglandins in coronary heart disease. Rationale for use of platelet-suppressive drugs. JAMA 249:2818–2823

73. Mehta P, Mehta J, Lawson D, Krop I, Letts LG (1986) Leukotrienes potentiale the effects of epinephrine and thrombin on human platelet aggregation. Thromb Res 41:731–738

74. Mehta J, Lopez LM, Wargovich T (1987) Eicosapentaenoic acid: Its relevance in atherosclerosis and coronary artery disease. Am J Cardiol 59:155–159

75. Miettinen TA, Naukkarinen V, Huttunen JK, Mattila S, Kumlin T (1982) Fatty-acid composition of serum lipids predicts myocardial infarction. Br Med J 285:993–996

76. Moncada S, Salmon JA (1986) Leukotrienes and tissue injury: The use of eicosapentaenoic acid in the control of white cell activation. Wiener Klin Wochenschrift 98:104–106

77. Mori TA, Codde JP, Vandongen R, Beilin LJ (1987) New findings in the fatty acid composition of individual platelet phospholipids in man after dietary fish oil supplementation. Lipids 22:744–750

78. Mullane KM, Read N, Salmon JA, Moncada S (1984) Role of leukocytes in acute myocardial infarction in anesthetized dogs: Relationship to myocardial salvage by antiinflammatory drugs. J Pharmacol Exp Ther 228:510–522

79. Murota S, Morita I (1985) Possible mechanisms of antithrombotic effect of eicosapentaenoic acid: Species specificity. Adv Prostagl Thrombox Leukot Res 15:257–259

80. Nathaniel DJ, Evans JF, Leblanc Y, Leveille C, Fitzsimmons BJ, Ford-Hutchinson AW (1985) Leukotriene A5 is a substrate and an inhibitor of rat and human neutrophil LTA4 hydrolase. Biochem Biophys Res Comm 131:827–835

81. Needleman P, Raz A, Minkes MS, Ferrendelli JA, Sprecher H (1979) Triene prostaglandins: prostacyclin and thromboxane biosynthesis and unique biological properties. Proc Natl Acad Sci USA 76:944–948

82. Needleman P, Turk J, Jakschik BA, Morrison AR, Lefkowith JB (1986) Arachidonate acid metabolism. Ann Rev Biochem 55:69–102

83. Nestel PJ, Connor WE, Reardon MF, Connor S, Wong S, Boston R (1984) Suppression by diets rich in fish oil of very low density lipoprotein production in man. J Clin Invest 74:82–89

84. Nestel PJ (1986) Fish oil attenuates the cholesterol induced rise in lipoprotein cholesterol. Am J Clin Nutr 43:752–757

85. Nestel PJ (1987) Polyunsaturated fatty acids. Am J Clin Nutr 45:1161–1167

86. Niewiarowski S, Rao AK (1983) Contribution of thrombogenic factors to the pathogenesis of atherosclerosis. Prog Cardiovasc Dis 26:197–222

87. Ochi K, Yoshimoto T, Yamamoto S, Taniguchi K, Miyamoto T (1983) Arachidonate-5-lipoxygenase of guinea pig peritoneal polymorphonuclear leukocytes: activation by adenosine 5'-triphosphate. J Biol Chem 258:5754–5758

88. Okegawa T, Jonas PE, DeSchryver K, Kawasaki A, Needleman P (1983) Metabolic and cellular alterations underlying the exaggerated renal prostaglandin and thromboxane synthesis in ureter obstruction in rabbits. Inflammatory response involving fibroblasts and mononuclear cells. J Clin Invest 71:81–90

89. Phillipson BR, Rothrock DW, Connor WE, Harris WS, Illingsworth DR (1985) Reduction of plasma lipids, lipoproteins, and apoproteins by dietary fish oils in patients with hypertriglyceridemia. N Engl J Med 312:1201–1216

90. Prescott SM (1984) The effect ofeicosapentaenoic acid on the leukotriene B production by human neutrophils. J Biol Chem 259:7615–7621

91. Prescott SM, Zimmermann GA, Morrison AR (1985) The effects of a diet rich in fish oil on human neutrophils: Identification of leukotriene B5 as a metabolite. Prostaglandins 30:209–227

92. Rao GHR, Radda E, White JG (1983) Effect of docosahexaenoic acid on arachidonic acid metabolism and platelet function. Biochem Biophys Res Commun 117:549–555

93. Riemersma RA, Wood DA, Butler EA (1986) Linoleic acid in adipose tissue and coronary heart disease. Br Med J 292:1423–1427

94. Rifkind BM (1986) Diet, plasma cholesterol, and coronary heart disease. J Nutr 116:1578–1580

95. Romson JL, Hook BG, Kunkel SL, Abrams JD, Schork MA, Lucchesi BR (1983) Reduction of the extent of ischemic myocardial injury by neutrophil depletion in the dog. Circulation 67:1016–1023

96. Ross R (1986) The pathogenesis of arteriosclerosis – an update. N Engl J Med 314:488–500

97. Sanders TAB, Naismith DJ, Haines AP, Vickers M (1980) Cod liver oil, platelet fatty acids, and bleeding time. Lancet 1:1189

98. Sanders TB, Vickers M, Haines AP (1981) Effect on blood lipids and hemostasis of a supplement of cod liver oil, rich in eicosapentaenoic and docosahexaenoic acids, in healthy young men. Clin Sci 61:317–324

99. Sanders TAB, Younger KM (1981) The effect of dietary supplements of omega-3 polyunsaturated fatty acids on the fatty acid composition of platelets and plasma choline phosphoglycerides. Br J Nutr 45:613–616

100. Sanders TAB (1987) Fish and coronary artery disease. Br Heart J 57:214–219

101. Saynor R, Verel D, Gillott T (1984) The long-term effect of dietary supplementation with fish lipid concentrate on serum lipids, bleeding time, platelets, and angina. Atherosclerosis 50:3–10

102. von Schacky C, Fischer S, Weber PC (1985) Long-term effects of dietary marine omega-3 fatty acids upon plasma and cellular lipids, platelet function, and eicosanoid formation in humans. J Clin Invest 76:1626–1631

103. von Schacky C, Weber PC (1985) Metabolism and effects on platelet function of the purified eicosapentaenoic and docosahexaenoic acids in humans. J Clin Invest 76:2446–2450

104. von Schacky C, Siess W, Fischer S, Weber PC (1985) A comparative study of eicosapentaenoic acid metabolism by human platelets in vivo and in vitro. J Lipid Res 26:457–464

105. Shea MJ, Driscoll RM, Romson JL, Bitt B, Lucchesi BR (1984) The beneficial effect of nafazatrom on experimental coronary thrombosis. Am Heart J 107:629–637

106. Schettler G (1986) Relevance of fatty acids and eicosanoids to clinical and preventive medicine. Prog Lipid Res 25:1–4

107. Schettler G (ed) (1987) Molecular biology of the arterial wall. Springer, Berlin Heidelberg New York

108. Shekelle RB, Missell L, Paul O, Shyrock A, Stammler J (1985) Fish consumption and mortality from coronary heart disease. N Engl J Med 313:820

109. Siess W, Scherer B, Böhling B, Roth P, Kurzmann I, Weber PC (1980) Platelet membrane fatty acids, platelet aggregation, and thromboxane formation during a mackerel diet. Lancet i:441–444

110. Simpson HCR, Barker K, Carter RD, Cassels E, Mann JI (1982) Low dietary intake of linoleic acid predisposes to myocardial infarction. Br Med J 285:683–684

111. Sinclair H, Gale M (1987) Eicosapentaenoic acid in fat. Lancet i:1202

112. Soter NA, Lewis RA, Corey EJ, Austen KF (1983) Local effects of synthetic leukotrienes in human skin. J Invest Dermatol 80:115–119

113. Strasser T, Fischer S, Weber PC (1985) Leukotriene B5 is formed in human neutrophils after dietary supplementation with icosapentaenoic acid. Proc Natl Acad Sci USA 82:1540–1543

114. Stubbs CD, Smith AD (1984) The modification of mammalian membrane polyunsaturated fatty acid composition in relation to membrane fluidity and function. Biochim Biophys Acta 779:89–137

115. Tamura Y, Hirai A, Terano T, Kumagai A, Yoshida S (1985) Effects of eicosapentaenoic acid on hemostatic function and serum lipids in humans. Adv Prostagl Thrombox Leukot Res 15:265–267

116. Terano T, Salmon JA, Moncada S (1984) Biosynthesis and biologic activity of leukotriene B5. Prostaglandins 27:217–232

117. Thorngren M, Gustafson A (1981) Effects of 11-week increase in dietary eicosapentaenoic acid on bleeding time, lipids, and platelet aggregation. Lancet ii:1190–1193
118. Thorogood M, Carter R, Benfield L, McPherson K, Mann JI (1987) Plasma lipids and lipoprotein cholesterol concentrations in people with different diets in Britain. Br Med J 295:351–357
119. Tripp CS, Unanue ER, Needleman P (1986) Monocyte migration explains the changes in macrophage arachidonate metabolism during the immue response. Proc Natl Acad Sci USA 83:9655–9659
120. Tzeng DY, Deuel TF, Huang JS, Baehner RL (1985) Platelet-derived growth factor promotes human peripheral monocyte activation. Blood 66:179–183
121. Wargovich T, Mehta J, Nichols WW, Pepine CJ, Conti CR (1985) Reduction of blood flow in normal and narrowed coronary arteries of dogs by leukotriene C. J Am Coll Cardiol 6:1047–1051
122. Weiner BH, Ockene IS, Jarmolych J, Fritz KE, Daoud AS (1985) Comparison of phatologic and angiographic findings in a porcine preparation of coronary athero-sclerosis. Circulation 72:1081–1086
123. Weiner BH, Ockene IS, Levine PH, Cuenoud HF, Fisher M, Johnson BF, Daoud AS, Jarmolych J, Hosmer D, Johnson MH, Natale A, Vaudreuil C, Hoogasian JJ (1986) Inhibition of atherosclerosis by cod-liver oil in a hyperlipidemic swine model. N Engl J Med 315:841–846
124. Weiner MA (1986) Cholesterol in foods rich in omega-3 fatty acid. N Engl J Med 315:833
125. Wong SH, Nestel PJ, Trimble RP, Storer GB, Illman RJ, Topping DL (1984) The adaptive effects of dietary fish and safflower oil on lipid and lipoprotein metabolism in perfused rat liver. Biochem. Biophys. Acta 792:103–109
126. Wood DA, Butler S, Riemersma RA, Thomson M, Oliver MF (1984) Adipose tissue and platelet fatty acids and coronary heart disease in Scottish men. Lancet ii:117–121
127. Wood DA, Riemersma RA, Butler S, Thomson M, MacIntyre C, Elton RA, Oliver MF (1987) Linoleic and eicosapentaenoic acids in adipose tissue and platelets and risk of coronary heart disease. Lancet i:177–183
128. Woodcock BE, Smith E, Lambert WH, Jones WM, Galloway JH, Greaves M, Preston FE (1984) Beneficial effect of fish oil on blood viscosity in peripheral vascular disease. Br Med J 288:592–594